Endocrinology:
Fast Focus Study Guide

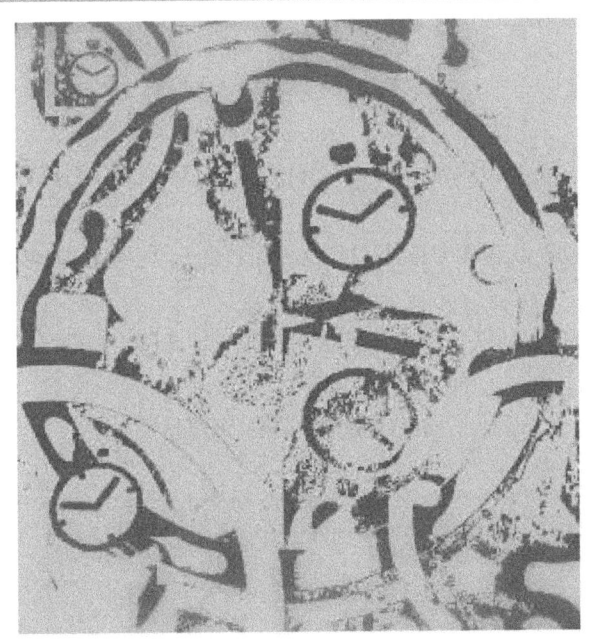

Acknowledgements

I dedicate this book to my beautiful
wife and children, who I love more
than all the water in all the oceans
and all the seas.

CONTENTS

- This book is written for any medical professionals who want to learn more about endocrinology.

- There are over 350 pages of easy to read facts about endocrinology.

- Put this book in your bathroom or on your coffee table.

- This is the perfect graduation gift for the aspiring physician or graduating physician.

- This Fast Focus Study Guide will provide you with a practical review of the key information you need to know.

- Buy this book now if you want this quick and concise information

Acromegaly is caused by sustained

release of growth hormone.

Growth hormone secreting tumor of the pituitary called somatotropinoma is the most common cause of acromegaly.

Insulin like growth factor I is secreted by the liver and to a lesser extent by other tissues in response to growth hormone and mediates several actions of growth hormone at the tissue level.

Bromocriptine is the primary non-surgical treatment of acromegaly. This drug decreases growth hormone levels in 75% of patients with acromegaly but is unlikely to totally normalize hormone levels.

There is an increased incidence of colon cancer among patients with acromegaly.

Acromegaly is an endocrine disorder characterized by hypertension secondary to expanded plasma volume, enlargement of the jaw and tongue, bony soft tissue overgrowth, coarsened facial features, laryngeal hypertrophy with secondary deepening of the voice.

Insulin like growth factor I is the preferred assay for acromegaly diagnosis.

Failure of growth hormone to suppress completely after 100 grams of glucose load and paradoxical growth hormone response to intravenous bolus of thyrotropin releasing hormone are two tests used to demonstrate abnormal growth hormone physiology.

2/3 of the time an ectopic ACTH producing tumor this is associated with oat cell tumors of lung.

Vasopressin and corticotropin releasing hormone are two positive effectors of ACTH.

ACTH is released in the anterior
pituitary and is regulated by cortisol

The common etiologies of adrenal insufficiency include autoimmune destruction of the adrenals; TB; Carcinomatous hemorrhage; Adrenal infarction; other (sarcoidosis, amyloidosis, fungal, post op).

Addisonian crisis is precipitated by stressors and is characterized by nausea/vomiting, diarrhea, abdominal pain, +/- fever, progressive lethargy, hypotension, and hypovolemic shock.

The classic triad of Addison's disease includes hyperkalemia, azotemia and hyponatremia.

Addison's disease is characterized by diarrhea with hyperpigmentation.

Approximately 80% of patients with Addison's disease have had autoimmune destruction of their adrenal glands.

Approximately 15% of patients with Addison's disease have had destruction of their adrenal glands related to tuberculosis infection.

Addisonian crisis is an acute
complication of adrenal insufficiency
characterized by circulatory collapse,
dehydration, nausea, vomiting,
hypoglycemia, and hyperkalemia.

Addison's disease is generalized
adrenal corticoid insufficiency.

Skin hyperpigmentation occurs in Addison's disease secondary to increased melanocyte stimulating hormone that occurs because of an increase of ACTH and a lack of negative feedback from cortisol.

The plasma cortisol is decreased in
patients with Addison's disease.

Adrenal adenoma or carcinoma result in a decreased plasma ACTH level.

The 5 major risk factors for adrenal
hemorrhage:
Post-operative state; Thromboembolic
disease; Sepsis; Hypotension;
Coagulopathy

Adrenal hyperplasia could result in an increase in the plasma ACTH.

The 17 hydroxyprogesterone level is the best screening test for congenital adrenal hyperplasia secondary to 11-hydroxylase deficiency or 21-hydroxylase deficiency.

Glucocorticoids; Mineralocorticoids; Adrenal androgens are three types of steroids produced from adrenal gland.

In primary insufficiency there is skin hyperpigmentation due to increased ACTH. In secondary adrenal insufficiency there is no hyperpigmentation because ACTH is decreased.

In primary adrenal disorder there is a combined mineralocorticoid and glucocorticoid deficiency. In secondary adrenal failure there is exogenous glucocorticoid suppression of the hypothalamic-pituitary-adrenal axis.

CMV, MAI, Cryptococcus, and Kaposi's sarcoma have all been implicated as common etiologies of adrenal insufficiency in patients with AIDS.

The cortrosyn stimulation test involves giving synthetic ACTH and then monitoring plasma levels of cortisol and aldosterone.

The cortrosyn stimulation test is done to differentiate the etiology of adrenal insufficiency

If the cortrosyn stimulation test is done on a patient with adrenal insufficiency because of intrinsic adrenal dysfunction there would be no rise in the cortisol level or the aldosterone level.

The tetrad of Conn's syndrome (hyperaldosteronism):

-Fatigue

-HTN

-HA

-Nocturia

Conn's syndrome is characterized by
hyperaldosteronism secondary to
abnormal secretion by adrenal
adenoma/carcinoma/hyperplasia, or
by ovarian tumor

Conn's syndrome is characterized by increased sodium, decreased potassium, increased urinary aldosterone, and low or normal serum renin levels

Hyperaldosteronism results in sodium and water retention with loss of potassium.

Conn's syndrome is characterized by hyper secretion of aldosterone from the zona glomerulosa of the adrenal gland resulting in hypokalemia, hypertension, and alkalosis

Secondary hyperaldosteronism is characterized by excessive aldosterone secretion from stimulation of the renin-angiotensin system Is associated with chronic liver disease, diuretics, pregnancy, renal artery stenosis, renin secreting neoplasm, Bartter' syndrome, hypovolemia, Na depletion, and malignant HTN

Turner's syndrome is the most

common cause of primary

amenorrhea

Primary amenorrhea is the absence of menarche after 16 years of age

ADH acts at the distal tubule and collecting duct to promote retention of free water to restore normal plasma osmolarity.

Antidiuretic hormone (ADH) is stimulated to be released by increased serum osmolality or decreased plasma volume.

Apoplexy is the disease characterized
by bleeding into a pituitary tumor
usually resulting in death

Calcitonin decreases serum calcium

and decreases serum PO4.

Calcitonin will cause the increased excretion of calcium at kidneys; Calcitonin will cause the increased PO4 reabsorption at kidneys

Calcitonin increased secondary to proliferation of Para follicular cells (C cells). This hormone lowers serum calcium and phosphate

Calcitonin will increase calcium

resorption at bones.

Calcitonin has no effect at intestines

11 B-hydroxylase deficiency is the second most common enzyme deficiency in congenital adrenal hyperplasia

21-hydroxylase deficiency and 11 B
hydroxylase deficiency are inherited
autosomal recessive.

In patients with 17 hydroxylase deficiency, 17 alpha-hydroxyprogesterone and progesterone are secreted in excess.

The most common cause of congenital adrenal hyperplasia is a deficiency in 21-hydroxylase.

In the cosyntropin stimulation test the cosyntropin, 250 micrograms, is given IV or IM, and plasma cortisol is measured 30 minutes later. The normal response is a stimulated plasma cortisol higher than 20 mug/dl (Clinical Endocrinology 44:147, 1996).

Elevated levels of 17-hydroxyprogesterone, androstenedione, and serum testosterone are the most common blood abnormalities seen in congenital adrenal hyperplasia

Endemic cretinism occurs because of lack of dietary iodine; sporadic cretinism occurs because of a defect in T4 formation.

The 24-hour urine cortisol is the most sensitive and specific test for hypercortisolism.

Cushing's disease is a disorder is characterized by excess production of ACTH by pituitary causing Cushing's syndrome

<5% of patients with Cushing's syndrome will have a negative dexamethasone suppression test.

Two sources for endogenous Cushing's syndrome include ACTH dependent pituitary or ectopic tumors and ACTH independent cortisol secreting adrenal tumors.

The dexamethasone suppression test

is done as a screening test for

Cushing's syndrome

<5% of patients with Cushing's syndrome will have a negative dexamethasone suppression test

Pituitary adenoma secreting ACTH is the most common cause of Cushing's syndrome.

You indirectly measure cortisol release by measuring the serum 17-hydroxycorticosteroid.

Approximately 20% of patients with Cushing's syndrome have diabetes.

The plasma cortisol is increased in patients with Cushing's syndrome.

There is lack of diurnal variation in
the plasma cortisol in patients with
Cushing's syndrome.

You would expect the serum sodium

to be increased in Cushing's

syndrome.

You would expect the serum potassium to be decreased in patients with Cushing's syndrome.

Approximately 50% of the time patients with Cushing's disease have normal plasma ACTH levels.

The corticotrophin releasing hormone stimulation test performed is done to evaluated increased and decreased cortisol levels.

The CRH stimulation test can help determine if Cushing's syndrome is related to a pituitary etiology or other cause.

Approximately 75% of patients with the pituitary adenomas will have a rise in the ACTH and cortisol levels.

Dawn phenomenon is a condition is characterized by hypoglycemia between 4am and 7am in absence of somogyi effect that occurs secondary to nocturnal release of growth hormones.

The drugs commonly associated with diabetes insipidus include lithium, cisplatin, amphotericin B, aminoglycosides, methoxyflurane, or demeclocycline.

After intranasal vasopressin (DDAVP) and careful water restriction, the urine osmolality will increase by at least 50% in patients with central diabetes insipidus.

The three most common symptoms in diabetes insipidus include polyuria, polydipsia and excessive thirst.

Deficiency of ADH is the cause of central diabetes insipidus

Nephrogenic diabetes insipidus is defined by ADH unresponsiveness? It is often acquired and results from drugs such as amphotericin B and lithium. It may also result from mechanisms secondary to parenchymal disease (HbS) or electrolyte dysfunction.

Diabetes insipidus is caused by a deficiency of ADH or a resistance to ADH leading to greater than 6 liters of urine per day with low urine concentration despite exam findings consistent with volume depletion

Neovascularization and vitreous
hemorrhage are two types of
proliferative diabetic retinopathy

Foot drop, hand muscle wasting, thigh muscle wasting and cranial nerve III, VI opthalmoplegia are four motor neuropathies secondary to diabetes mellitus

Name 5 manifestations of diabetic neuropathy include symmetric proximal motor neuropathy, symmetric distal sensory polyneuropathy, focal motor neuropathy, autonomic neuropathy and acute painful neuropathy.

Cushing's syndrome, acromegaly, glucagonoma, and pheochromocytoma are four hormonal excesses can result in diabetes.

Three drugs associated with the development of diabetes include glucocorticoids, diuretics and oral contraceptives

Hyperlipidemia, myotonic dystrophy and hemochromatosis are three genetic syndromes have commonly been associated with diabetes.

Neurogenic bladder and impotence are two GU disturbances of diabetes mellitus.

Age 15 is the peak age of incidence of type I diabetes mellitus.

The hemoglobin A1C a marker for mean blood glucose over 60-120 days

90% of diabetics in the western word

have type II DM.

Infection is the most common precipitating factor for hyperosmolar coma in type II diabetics.

Islet cell antibody found in 90% of patients within first year of diagnosis of type I diabetes mellitus.

About 30% of patients with

gestational diabetes will develop

DM within 5 years

Type II diabetes mellitus is characterized by 90% concordance in identical twins and is increased with obesity.

Hemolysis of the red cells with falsely decrease the hemoglobin.

A1C

Renal failure will falsely decrease the hemoglobin A1C because of decreased red cell survival time.

Thalassemia will falsely increase the hemoglobin A1C because of increases in the fetal hemoglobin.

The formula used to calculate an estimated mean glucose concentration for a hemoglobin A1C is:

Mean blood glucose = 33.3(HbA1c) − 86

Hemoglobin A1C is not a good screening test for diabetes. It currently is utilized to determine an estimate of chronic blood glucose levels in patients known to have diabetes.

The C-peptide level is expected to
be elevated in patients with
insulinoma

Concordance is seen in 50% of identical twins with type I diabetes mellitus.

The beta-hydroxybutyrate test is often done to evaluate and monitor patients with ketoacidosis.

The most common neuropathy seen with diabetes mellitus is peripheral symmetrical sensorimotor neuropathy associated with a stocking and glove distribution.

The free thyroxin index (FTI) corrects for any abnormal T4 values related to protein binding. It is calculated with the following formula:

FTI = T4 x T3RU / 100; Normal values are 2-5

Men can rarely have galactorrhea secondary to a prolactinoma. The most common symptoms of hyperprolactinemia in men include hypogonadism, depressed FSH and LH and depressed testosterone.

A woman with hypothyroidism have can have galactorrhea secondary to the lack of feedback from the thyroid gland to the hypothalamus leads to elevation of TRH, which is a positive modulator for prolactin release.

If medications are not the etiology of galactorrhea then MRI imaging of the pituitary gland should be done.

Prolactinomas are the most common pituitary adenoma, comprising approximately 25-40% of cases.

The most common cause of

hyperthyroidism is Grave's disease.

The three characteristic findings in Grave's disease include diffuse goiter with high uptake for I-131, ophthalmopathy and thyroid dermopathy (pretibial myxedema)

Grave's disease is associated with infiltrative ophthalmopathy, infiltrative dermopathy (pretibial myxedema is raised hyper pigmented areas of pretibial region and feet), and thyroid acropachy (clubbing of fingers associated with periosteal new bone formation in other areas)

Graves disease is characterized by IgG antibodies to TSH receptors on thyroid cells which stimulates thyroid cell growth and synthesis and release of thyroid hormones

Grave's disease can present with exophthalmos.

Grave's disease is caused by thyroid stimulating antibodies which activate thyroid adenylate cyclase and compete with TSH for receptors on thyroid cell membranes

In the third trimester of pregnancy, Graves disease is treated with propylthiouracil. In the second trimester, subtotal thyroidectomy is the therapy of choice.

Insulin-like growth factor mediates the trophic changes of growth hormone

Zollinger Ellison can be treated with excision of tumor, parietal cell vagotomy, or total gastrectomy.

Gynecomastia is evaluated by taking a drug history, thorough physical exam with measurement of testes, evaluation of liver tests, serum androsenedione, plasma estradiol, HCG, LH, and testosterone.

Estrogen mediates the growth of

breast tissue in men

Cimetidine and spironolactone interfere with binding of testosterone to the receptor and can cause gynecomastia.

If the work up of gynecomastia reveals an increased LH and a depressed testosterone the cause is most likely testicular failure.

If the work up for gynecomastia reveals depressed LH and depressed testosterone, the most likely etiology is most likely primary estrogen production is likely the etiology (this can occur in the setting of sertoli cell tumor)

If both the testosterone and LH are elevated in the setting of gynecomastia, then the most likely etiology is androgen resistance or gonadotropin secreting tumor.

The physical exam findings of the goiter associated with Hashimoto's thyroiditis is typically have a painless goiter which is firm or hard to palpation often involving the pyramidal lobe of the thyroid.

Antibodies to thyroglobulin, thyroid peroxidase, or the sodium-iodide symporter are seen in 90% of patients with Hashimoto's thyroiditis.

Hashimoto's thyroiditis usually results in permanent hypothyroidism, however there have been reports of rare remissions resulting decreased need for thyroid supplements.

There is a 4% annual risk of developing clinical hypothyroidism in patients with subclinical hypothyroidism with a positive anti-thyroid peroxidase antibodies.

The symptoms of hypothyroidism are non-specific and no specific symptom is diagnostic of hypothyroidism. These symptoms include, but are not limited to weight gain, fatigue, dry skin, puffy face, brittle hair, hair loss, constipation, decreased libido, bradycardia, and loss of memory.

Hashimoto's thyroiditis is the autoimmune disease involving a defect of suppressor T-lymphocytes with progressive destruction of the thyroid gland by an inflammatory process associated with the presence of anti-mitochondrial antibodies is present (>90%).

There is a 60-fold increase in risk of
thyroid lymphoma following
Hashimoto's thyroiditis.

Hashimoto's thyroiditis is the most common cause of hypothyroidism in the US

Hypothyroidism due to thyroid failure in patients with Hashimoto's thyroiditis is due to autoimmune destruction of the thyroid gland.

Hashimoto's thyroiditis is often associated with development of a goiter, but a goiter is not always present.

Hashimoto's thyroiditis can be separated into those with atrophic autoimmune thyroiditis and goitrous autoimmune thyroiditis

Hashimoto's thyroiditis is more common in women with a ratio of women to men of (7:1)

Hashimoto's thyroiditis is most commonly associated with hypothyroidism, however patients will rarely have short episodes of transient hyperthyroidism associated with inflammation and thyroid follicular disruption.

There is a 30-60% concordance of Hashimoto's thyroiditis in monozygotic twins.

Hashimoto's thyroiditis is seen at increased rates in people with Down's syndrome and Turner's syndrome.

Hashimoto's thyroiditis is seen later in life in about 20% of patients with a history of transient postpartum thyroiditis.

Increased HbF, chronic renal failure, splenectomy, dialysis, thalassemia, and increased triglycerides can increase the HbA1C

DHEA-S produced in the adrenal glands.

DHEA-S is measured to determine if the
adrenal glands are producing androgens

DHEA-S is often measured in the

evaluation of hirsutism

Peripheral tissue can metabolize
DHEA-S produced in the adrenal
glands into androgens and estrogen

Stein-Leventhal Syndrome is the most common hormonal cause of hirsutism in women.

Frontal balding, clitoromegaly, deepening of voice, acne, and increase shoulder girdle muscles are 5 signs of female virilization.

Decrease in breast size, amenorrhea, and loss of body contours are 3 signs of defeminization.

21-hydroxylase deficiency is the most common etiology of congenital adrenal hyperplasia however rarely a 11-hydroxylase deficiency is identified.

Polycystic ovary disease is characterized by hirsutism, obesity, amenorrhea, and large cystic ovaries

Cushing's syndrome can develop secondary to production of corticotropin from an adrenal adenoma, pituitary tumor, adrenal carcinoma, or ectopic secretion of corticotropin.

Ovarian sources of androgen excess usually present with elevated levels of testosterone, whereas DHEAS is usually elevated in adrenal sources.

Measurement of serum aldosterone is often done to evaluate for hyperaldosteronism in patients with hypertension.

The serum renin be depressed in patients with primary hyperaldosteronism.

An aldosterone producing adenoma is the most common cause of primary hyperaldosteronism.

Bilateral adrenal hyperplasia will be seen in about 30% of patients with primary hyperaldosteronism.

Secondary aldosteronism can be seen in patients with cirrhosis, renal failure, and cardiac failure.

Hyporeninemic hypoaldosteronism is the most common cause of secondary hypoaldosteronism

Heparin induced hyperkalemia

can be seen in as much as 7% of

patients on a heparin drip

Calcitonin results in the inhibition of

osteoclasts (bone resorption).

Serum calcitonin is most often performed to diagnose and follow medullary thyroid carcinoma.

The ionized calcium measures the
amount of calcium circulating
unbound (free) in the circulation

Acidosis results in increased free

calcium in circulation

Alkalosis results in decreased free

calcium in circulation

Air bubbles in a sample used to measure ionized calcium will result in decrease CO_2 concentration and increased pH (alkalosis) resulting in a false decrease in the measured ionized calcium.

Primary hyperparathyroidism is the most common cause of asymptomatic hypercalcemia.

Osteitis fibrosa cystica is associated with hypercalcemia is characterized by bone pain, fractures, deformities, bone cysts, sub periosteal bone resorption in the phalanges, and generalized osteopenia

Four secondary causes of hyperprolactinemia include prescribed and recreational drug use, hypothyroidism, chronic renal failure and pregnancy.

In SIADH the Urine osmolality is higher than plasma osmolality because of the inability to concentrate urine maximally even in the presence of hyponatremia.

Primary hyperparathyroidism is
characterized by increased secretion
of PTH by parathyroid glands

Secondary hyperparathyroidism is characterized by increased secretion of PTH from the parathyroid secondary to renal failure and constant calcium wasting.

Tertiary hyperparathyroidism is characterized by persistent increase of increased release of PTH secondary to refractory hyperplasia caused by secondary hyperparathyroidism. So after the calcium is corrected, the calcium fails to regulate the PTH secretion

Vit D action at bone---increase Ca resorption; Vit D action at kidney---increase Ca resorption; Vit D action at intestine----increase Ca resorption and PO4 resorption

Hyporeninemic hypoaldosteronism (decreased aldosterone secondary to decreased renin can be seen in the setting of renal disease secondary to various factors) and in the setting of aldosterone deficiency (found associated with deficiency of other adrenal glucocorticoid hormones).

Zollinger Ellison is diagnosed with the fasting serum gastrin level and the secretin stimulation test.

47% of the circulating calcium circulates unbound (free) in the circulation

Approximately 1/3 of gastrinomas are metastatic at diagnosis.

Only 10-20% of thyroid nodules are malignant.

MEN I is associated with about 20%
of patients diagnosed with Zollinger-
Ellison syndrome.

Approximately 80% of the time an
increased cortisol will be related to an
ACTH dependent etiology

Approximately 90% of patients with Zollinger-Ellison will also have peptic ulcer diseases

In correcting SIADH with hyponatremia, saline should be given with a loop diuretic because the loop diuretic facilitates the free water excretion.

In hypoparathyroidism the serum calcium is decreased, the serum PO4 is increased and the alkaline phosphatase is normal.

The plasma cortisol increased in the setting of ectopic ACTH production.

The plasma cortisol increased in the setting of ectopic ACTH production.

Nine causes of thyrotoxicosis include Grave's disease; Toxic multinodular goiter; Thyroiditis; Iodine-induced hyperthyroidism; factitious thyrotoxicosis; Secondary to excessive TSH; Toxic thyroid carcinoma; Toxic struma ovarii.

Bromocriptine (dopamine agonist) is one therapeutic option for treatment of prolactinomas.

Seven symptoms of a thyroid storm include fever> 100'F; Marked anxiety, agitation, psychosis; Hyperhidrosis, heat intolerance; Weakness, muscle wasting; Tachydysrhythmias, palpitations; Diarrhea, nausea, vomiting; Elderly patients have tachycardia, CHF, and mental status changes.

Two diagnostic hallmarks of primary hyperparathyroidism include Hypercalcemia; Increased PTH concentration (Primary hyperparathyroidism is most commonly due to parathyroid adenoma).

Phentolamine, prazosin; and phenoxybenamine are three anti-hypertensive medications commonly used in patients with pheochromocytoma prior to surgery.

Three vascular causes of hyopituaritism include post-partum necrosis (Sheehan's syndrome); Hemorrhagic infarction of pituitary tumor and aneurysm of carotid artery.

Hashimoto's thyroiditis and idiopathic myxedema are two autoimmune causes of hypothyroidism?

Pemberton's sign is facial redness and choking when arms are extended above the head in patients with sub sternal goiters.

The morning levels of ACTH are generally about 2x higher than the levels of ACTH in the evening.

Reverse T3 is the measurement of the percentage of labeled T3 bound to the resin after being exposed to test serum thyroid binding globulin. If the thyroid binding globulin is increased then a smaller percentage of the labeled T3 will bind to the resin

MEN I is characterized by tumors of the parathyroid (90% have hyperplasia), pancreas (66% have islet cell tumors, 50% have Zollinger Ellison, 20% have Insulinoma), and pituitary 66%.

Signs of hypothyroidism include dry, cold, thick skin, periorbital edema, slow speech, vitiligo, coarse, thin hair, HTN, ascites, pallor of skin, bradycardia, and thick tongue.

The 4 types of thyroid carcinoma include papillary (60%), follicular (20%), medullary (10%); and anaplastic (10%).

The 5 H's of pheochromocytoma are headache, HTN, hyperhidrosis, hyperglycemia, and hyper metabolism.

The components of MEN IIB include mucosal neuromas, medullary thyroid carcinoma, marfanoid body habitus, and pheochromocytoma.

The conditions associated with increased ionized calcium include hyperparathyroidism, malignancy, ectopic PTH production, and vitamin D excess.

The four pituitary hormones and the effect of their absence in hypopituitarism include growth hormone deficiency (no manifestations in adults), gonadal dysfunction (amenorrhea, impotence, hypogonadotropic hypogonadism), hypothyroidism; and ACTH deficiency (develops in late stages, can manifest as Addisonian crisis).

Growth hormone and prolactin deficiency are most commonly seen at presentation in patients with Sheehan's syndrome.

Impotence and menstrual abnormalities are the most common symptoms of hyperprolactinemia in men and women.

Abdominal pain and diarrhea are the most common symptoms of Zollinger Ellison syndrome.

The parameters of MEN IIA include medullary thyroid carcinoma, pheochromocytoma and hyperparathyroidism.

Thyroid nodules are more likely to be malignant if they are in patients with a history of radiation to the neck, are rapidly growing, occur in young men, appears cold on a radioactive iodine scintiscan, or appear solid on ultrasound.

The six major hormones secreted by the pituitary gland include growth hormone, prolactin, and luteinizing hormone, follicle stimulating hormone, thyroid stimulating hormone, and adrenocorticotropic hormone.

Increased calcium reabsorption, increased PO4 excretion and increased conversion of vitamin D to active form are the three actions of PTH at the kidney.

Alimentary form, early type II diabetes, and idiopathic are the three forms of hypoglycemia.

PTH increases calcium reabsorption

and increased PO4 reabsorption.

The two main sources of SIADH include the lung (small cell lung cancer, pneumonia, increased PEEP) and CNS (trauma, CVA, anesthesia, morphine).

The two secondary causes of hypothyroidism include hypothalamic dysfunction (irradiation, granulomatous disease, neoplasms) and pituitary dysfunction (irradiation, surgery on pituitary, idiopathic hypopituitarism, neoplasm, and post-partum pituitary necrosis).

Hyperprolactinemia is associated with oligomenorrhea or amenorrhea in females.

The three benign lesions of the thyroid include adenomatous goiter, follicular adenoma, and hyper functioning adenoma.

Three common findings of subacute thyroiditis include fever, thyroid tenderness, and thyrotoxicosis.

Three causes of primary hyperparathyroidism include adenoma (85%), hyperplasia (15%), and carcinoma (1%).

Three findings that characterize Sipple's syndrome include medullary carcinoma of the thyroid, pheochromocytoma, and hyperparathyroidism.

Three neuroendocrine effects of morphine include increased release of prolactin, increased release of growth hormone, and inhibition of GNRH release.

In hyperparathyroidism in renal disease there is increased phosphorus secondary to decreased phosphorus excretion; There is decreased Ca because of decreased renal synthesis of 1, 25 Vit D; There is increased PTH because of the increased serum phosphorus and decreased serum calcium.

Two infiltrative causes of
hypopituitarism include
hemochromatosis and histiocytosis X.

Osteitis fibrosa cystica is associated with hypercalcemia is characterized by bone pain, fractures, deformities, bone cysts, sub periosteal bone resorption in the phalanges, and generalized osteopenia.

Hypogonadotropic hypogonadism is characterized by low gonadotropin levels and impaired testicular function as a result of injury to the pituitary or hypothalamus.

Euthyroid sick syndrome is characterized by low thyroxin (T4), Low TSH, and a high reverse T3

Nelson's syndrome is characterized by hyperpigmentation, headache, exophthalmos, increased sex hormones, and pituitary enlargement and visual field defects.

MEN I typically involves the
pituitary, pancreas, and the
parathyroid.

MEN I (parathyroid, pancreas, pituitary) must be ruled out in patients with Zollinger-Ellison syndrome.

The diagnosis of hyperparathyroidism is suggested when there is an increased calcium, increased PTH, decreased phosphorus, and increased chloride.

Hashimoto's disease is characterized by the presence of antithyroid antibodies.

Sheehan's syndrome is characterized by postpartum necrosis of the pituitary gland.

MEN II (almost all of these will be bilateral) must be ruled out in a patient with pheochromocytoma.

Hyperprolactinemia is associated with tricyclic antidepressants, phenothiazines, butyrephenones, metoclopramide, reserpine, alpha-methyldopa and cimetidine.

Brown tumor is a giant cell tumor found in osteitis fibrosa cystica and occurs secondary to hyperparathyroidism.

In factitious hypoglycemia that occurs when patients take oral drugs that promote insulin release the C-peptide levels will be increased, reflecting the endogenous insulin release. These patients can be screened for oral hypoglycemic medications which should show up in their serum or urine.

A common site of extra-adrenal pheochromocytomas are the organs of Zuckerman (Embryonic chromaffin cells around the abdominal aorta that normally atrophy during childhood).

The C-peptide connects the A and B portions of the insulin molecule.

There is a theoretical risk that B-blockers can delay recovery from hypoglycemia. Clinically this is likely not significant.

80% of insulinomas are benign
solitary adenomas.

PTH increases calcium absorption via

vitamin D.

Headache, palpitations, and episodic diaphoresis is the classic triad of pheochromocytoma.

Acute thyroiditis occurs secondary to bacterial thyroid infection.

Subacute thyroiditis occurs post upper respiratory virus.

Chronic thyroiditis is also known as Hashimoto's thyroiditis.

A Hot thyroid nodule is characterized by increased I-131 uptake and is seen as a functioning or hyper functioning nodule.

Cold thyroid nodules are characterized by decreased I-131 uptake and are considered a non-functioning nodule.

Increased total serum thyroxine (T4) is the effect of pregnancy on the laboratory measurement of thyroid function.

Vitamin D deficiency is characterized by decreased calcium, decreased serum PO4, and increased alkaline phosphatase.

80% of circulating T3 is derived from de-iodination of circulating T4.

The etiology of hypoglycemia in a patient with elevated insulin levels and relatively decreased C-peptide levels is exogenous insulin administration.

The initial treatment of primary hyperparathyroidism is aimed at treatment of the resulting hypercalcemia and includes intravenous fluids until volume status is returned to euvolemic state, followed by furosemide (no thiazides).

The major binding protein for circulating T3 and T4 is thyroid-binding globulin, which has 10 times the affinity for T4 than for T3.

Propylthiouracil (PTU) prevents
conversion of T4 to T3 by inhibiting
thyroid peroxidase.

Diazoxide suppresses insulin secretion and is the medical treatment for insulinoma.

ACTH independent increases in cortisol are most commonly related to adrenal carcinoma or adrenal adenoma.

Pituitary adenoma is the most common cause of an ACTH dependent increase in cortisol.

Primary hyperparathyroidism is the most common cause of asymptomatic hypercalcemia.

Small cell lung cancer is the most common cause of ectopic ACTH production.

Hashimotos thyroiditis is the most common cause of goiter and hypothyroidism in the adult.

Thyroid surgery is the most common cause of hypoparathyroidism.

Sheehan's syndrome is the most common cause of hypopituitarism worldwide.

Gastrinomas most commonly
metastasize to the liver.

The medical management of Zollinger Ellison syndrome most commonly involves the administration of proton pump inhibitors to block the secretion of gastric acid from the gastrinoma.

Hyperparathyroidism is the most common presenting symptom of MEN I.

Myxedema coma secondary to hypothyroidism is a life threatening complication of hypothyroidism is characterized by profound lethargy or coma

Serum calcitonin is most often performed to diagnose and follow medullary thyroid carcinoma

Papillary thyroid carcinoma (women in 2nd and 3rd decade of life, Psammoma bodies, spread by lymphatics and local invasion) is the most common type of thyroid carcinoma

Zollinger Ellison is associated with a 40% 5-year survival after total gastrectomy

The rule of '10' for pheochromocytoma; 10% extra renal; 10% malignant; 10% familial; 10% children; 10% bilateral; 10% are multiple.

A micro adenoma of the pituitary
gland is < 1 cm in size.

Nelson's syndrome is the syndrome characterized by the presence of a pituitary adenoma in a patient who has undergone bilateral adrenalectomy

Whipples Triad is characterized by hypoglycemia secondary to fasting; Glucose < 50 during symptoms. Patients have relief of symptoms with administration of glucose.

Zollinger Ellison syndrome is caused by a tumor producing gastrin (gastrinoma) which results in increased production of gastric acid resulting in peptic ulcers and diarrhea

The somatostatin receptor
scintigraphy with 111-In-pentetreotide
and SPECT is usually the first test
done to locate a gastrinoma.

A urinary sulfonylurea measurement and C-peptide levels can be done to rule out a factitious hypoglycemia.

Three findings associated with
MEN II (Sipple's syndrome)
include medullary thyroid
carcinoma, pheochromocytoma,
and hyperparathyroidism.

Three findings are associated with MEN III include medullary thyroid carcinoma, pheochromocytoma, and multiple mucosal neuromas.

Patients with ectopic ACTH production (i.e. from SCLC) will have no change in the cortisol or ACTH levels in response to a CRH stimulation test.

Patients in thyrotoxicosis will have an increased serum T4 and T3 and a decreased TSH.

Parathyroid damage after thyroidectomy is characterized by decreased serum calcium and increased phosphorus.

An ionized calcium would be the test of choice after multiple transfusions containing citrate, in patients with hepatic dysfunction, renal failure, critical illness, and in patients with known hyperparathyroidism with a normal total calcium

Calcitonin is produced and excreted

by the thyroid C cells.

Grave's disease is almost always associated with hyperthyroidism of pregnancy.

Zollinger Ellison is characterized by recurrent peptic ulcers in unusual locations, diarrhea, hypercalcemia, renal stones, and a family history of endocrine tumors

Hyperthyroidism is characterized by diarrhea with goiter, tremor, and tachycardia.

Propylthiouracil works by inhibiting thyroid peroxidase and thereby decreasing the synthesis of thyroid hormones as well and by preventing the conversion of T4 to T3.

Subacute (viral) thyroiditis is a form of hyperthyroidism will generally follow a viral illness. It is characterized by mild to moderate hyperthyroidism and a mildly enlarged and tender thyroid gland.

Pituitary hormone deficiency can result in growth hormone deficiency, hypothydoidism, or ACTH deficiency.

Somatostatin inhibits growth hormone secretion, inhibits secretion of insulin and glucagon, and can reduce fasting hyperglycemia in insulin dependent diabetics by suppression of glucagon secretion.

The free thyroxine index will give the most accurate evaluation of thyroid status.

MEN II is characterized by medullary thyroid carcinoma, pheochromocytoma, and hyperpigmentation.

The inferior thyroid artery supplies all four parathyroid glands.

Polyuria, polydipsia, and excessive thirst are the three most common symptoms in diabetes insipidus.

Signs and symptoms of a thyroid nodule that suggests carcinoma includes elevated calcitonin, history of rapid development, vocal cord paralysis, history of radiation to neck, cervical adenopathy, and a hard fixed mass

Papillary thyroid carcinoma has

Psammoma bodies.

It imperative to give IV fluids with the insulin in the setting of hyperglycemic, hyperosmolar, non-ketotic coma because if no IV fluids are given, the patient can become hypotensive as the glucose shifts from the extracellular to the intracellular space resulting in a net fluid shift into cells.

Zollinger Ellison associated with MEN I is most often characterized by multifocal disease. Because of this, it is difficult to surgically resect all of the gastrinomas.

In SIADH, elevated ADH leads to hyponatremia only if water intake exceeds excretion.

NSAIDS should be discontinued
when treating SIADH because
NSAIDS potentiate the effect of ADH
by blocking prostaglandin synthesis.

The C-peptide is generally measured when there is a question between factitious hypoglycemia and insulinoma.

You would not use aspirin during a thyroid storm because it displaces thyroid hormone from its binding protein.

Reidel's thyroiditis is characterized by extensive fibrosis of the thyroid resulting in a hard woody thyroid.

Foot drop, hand muscle wasting, thigh muscle wasting, and cranial nerve III and VI ophthalmoplegia are four motor neuropathies that can develop secondary to diabetes mellitus.

Glucocorticoids, mineralocorticoids, and adrenal androgens are steroids produced from adrenal gland.

Serum calcitonin is most often performed to diagnose and follow medullary thyroid carcinoma.

Hyperparathyroidism in renal disease occurs because there is increased phosphorus secondary to decreased phosphorus excretion, there is decreased Ca because of decreased renal synthesis of 1, 25 Vit D, and there is increased PTH because of the increased serum phosphorus and decreased serum calcium.

Primary hyperparathyroidism is characterized by hypercalcemia and increased PTH concentration.

Tertiary hyperparathyroidism is characterized by a persistent increased release of PTH secondary to refractory hyperplasia caused by secondary hyperparathyroidism.

The alpha and beta subunits of insulin are cleaved from pro-insulin in the beta cell and released in equimolar amounts with the C-peptide.

11 Beta-hydroxylase deficiency is the second most common enzyme deficiency in congenital adrenal hyperplasia.

17 alpha-hydroxyprogesterone and progesterone are the steroids secreted in excess secondary to buildup proximal to the block in patients with 17 hydroxylase deficiency.

21-hydroxylase deficiency and 11 B-hydroxylase deficiency are inherited autosomal recessive.

47% of the circulating calcium circulates unbound (free) in the circulation.

A woman with hypothyroidism could develop galactorrhea because the lack of feedback from the thyroid gland to the hypothalamus. This could result in elevation of TRH, which is a positive modulator for prolactin release.

Addisonian crisis is precipitated by stressors and is characterized by nausea/vomiting, diarrhea, abdominal pain, +/- fever, progressive lethargy, hypotension, and hypovolemic shock (will have decreased sodium and increased potassium secondary to absence.

Adrenal function can be suppressed in patients with a long history of uncorrected primary hypothyroidism. In these patients acute adrenal insufficiency can occur with initiating thyroid replacement.

Antibodies to thyroglobulin, thyroid peroxidase, or the sodium-iodide symporter are seen in 90% of patients with Hashimoto's thyroiditis.

Approximately 15% of patients with Addison's disease have had destruction of their adrenal glands related to tuberculosis infection.

Bromocriptine decreases growth hormone levels in 75% of patients with acromegaly but is unlikely to totally normalize hormone levels

Calcitonin results in the inhibition of osteoclasts (bone resorption).

Calcitonin will cause the increased excretion of calcium and increased PO4 reabsorption at kidneys.

Calcium channel blockers in patients with diabetes provide pressure reduction without adverse effects on lipids, glucose, or autonomic function.

Classic triad of pheochromocytoma:-
Headache-Palpitations-Episodic
diaphoresis

Decreased testosterone production or testosterone action, increased estrogen, and drugs are the three mechanisms of pathologic gynecomastia.

Endemic cretinism occurs because of lack of dietary iodine. Sporadic cretinism occurs because of a defect in T4 formation.

Graves disease is characterized by Infiltrative ophthalmopathy, infiltrative dermopathy (pretibial myxedema is raised hyper pigmented areas of pretibial region and feet), or thyroid acropachy (clubbing of fingers associated with periosteal new bone formation.

Hashimoto's thyroiditis is most commonly associated with hypothyroidism, however patients will rarely have short episodes of transient hyperthyroidism associated with inflammation and thyroid follicular disruption.

Hashimoto's thyroiditis usually results in permanent hypothyroidism, however there have been reports of rare remissions resulting decreased need for thyroid supplements.

Hemoglobin A1C can be falsely increased by elevated HbF, chronic renal failure, splenectomy, dialysis, thalassemia, or increased triglycerides.

Hirsutism can be associated with either defeminization (decreased estrogen) or virilization (increased testosterone). The 3 signs of defeminization are decrease in breast size, amenorrhea, and loss of body contours.

Hyperkalemia, azotemia, and hyponatremia is the classic triad of Addison's disease.

Hyperparathyroidism, malignancy, ectopic PTH production, and vitamin D excess are all associated with hypercalcemia.

Hypoaldosteronism can develop because of hyporeninemic hypoaldosteronism (decreased aldosterone secondary to decreased renin. typical of renal disease secondary to various factors) or because of aldosterone deficiency.

Hypoaldosteronism is a common problem in the diabetic that is manifested by hyperkalemia that is typically mild and out of proportion to accompanying azotemia.

Hypogonadism, depressed FSH and LH, and depressed testosterone are the more common findings of hyperprolactinemia in men.

Hypothyroidism due to thyroid failure in patients with Hashimoto's thyroiditis is due to autoimmune destruction of the thyroid gland.

Hypothyroidism is characterized by periorbital edema, slow speech, vitiligo, coarse hair, hypertension, ascites, pallor, bradycardia, thick tongue and dry, cold, thick skin.

If no IV fluids are given to patients with hyperglycemic hyperosmolar non-ketotic coma, the patient can become hypotensive as the glucose shifts from the extracellular to the intracellular space resulting in a net fluid shift into cells.

In primary adrenal failure there is a combined mineralocorticoid and glucocorticoid deficiency. In secondary adrenal failure there is exogenous glucocorticoid suppression of the hypothalamic-pituitary-adrenal axis.

In primary adrenal insufficiency skin hyperpigmentation develops due to increased ACTH. In secondary adrenal insufficiency there is no skin hyperpigmentation because ACTH is decreased.

In the third trimester of pregnancy, Graves disease is treated with Propylthiouracil. In the second trimester, subtotal thyroidectomy is the therapy of choice.

Inadequate dexamethasone suppression is suggestive of Cushing's syndrome, but as much as 30% of patients with a positive test do not have Cushing's syndrome.

Intranasal vasopressin (DDAVP) and careful water restriction will result in an increase in urine osmolality by at least 50% in patients with central diabetes insipidus.

Medullary carcinoma is associated
with MEN II.

Nelson's syndrome is found in patients with Cushings after an adrenalectomy and is characterized by hyperpigmentation, headache, exophthalmos, increased sex hormones, pituitary enlargement and visual field defects.

Neovascularization and vitreous hemorrhage are two types of proliferative diabetic retinopathy.

Ovarian sources of androgen excess usually present with elevated levels of testosterone. Adrenal sources of androgen excess usually are associated with elevations of DHEAS.

Patients with Hashimoto's thyroiditis typically have a firm, painless goiter, often involving the pyramidal lobe of the thyroid.

Polyuria, polydipsia, and excessive thirst are the three most common symptoms in diabetes insipidus.

Pituitary hormone deficiency can result in growth hormone deficiency, hypothyroidism, or ACTH deficiency.

Primary (Addison's) adrenal insufficiency is associated with skin hyperpigmentation due to increased ACTH.

Secondary adrenal insufficiency has no hyperpigmentation because ACTH is decreased.

PTH functions at the kidney to increase calcium reabsorption, increases PO4 excretion, and increase conversion of vitamin D to active form.

Skin hyperpigmentation in patients with adrenal insufficiency occurs because of increased melanocyte stimulating hormone that results from an increase of ACTH and a lack of negative feedback from cortisol.

The beta -hydroxybutyrate test is often done to evaluate and monitor patients with ketoacidosis.

The ionized calcium measures the amount of calcium circulating unbound (free) in the circulation.

The most common type of ectopic

ACTH producing tumor are oat cell

tumors of lung.

The most common type of thyroid
carcinoma is papillary thyroid
carcinoma. It is most commonly seen
in women in their 2nd and 3rd decade
of life and is characterized by
Psammoma bodies

The secondary causes of hypothyroidism include hypothalamic dysfunction (irradiation, granulomatous disease, neoplasms), and pituitary dysfunction (irradiation, surgery on pituitary, idiopathic hypopit, neoplasm, post-partum pituitary necrosis).

The serum glucose in patients with hyperosmolar hyperglycemia should be lowered at no more than 100 mg/dl/hour because cerebral and pulmonary edema can develop if lowered too quickly.

The signs of thyrotoxicosis are thyroid enlargement, lid lag, opthalmoplegia, proptosis, warm smooth skin, pretibial myxedema, fine tremor, brisk reflexes, onycholysis, and tachycardia or A-fib.

There is a 4% annual risk of developing clinical hypothyroidism in patients with subclinical hypothyroidism with a positive anti-thyroid peroxidase antibodies.

The secondary causes of hypothyroidism include hypothalamic dysfunction (irradiation, granulomatous disease, neoplasms), and pituitary dysfunction (irradiation, surgery on pituitary, idiopathic hypo pit, neoplasm, post-partum pituitary necrosis).

Thyroid nodules are more likely to be malignant if they are in patients with a history of radiation to the neck, are rapidly growing, occur in young men, appear cold on a radioactive iodine scintiscan, or appear solid on ultrasound.

Urine osmolality is higher than plasma osmolality in SIADH because of the inability to concentrate urine maximally even in the presence of hyponatremia.

This concludes 650 Pages of Facts Every Medical Student, Resident, and Physician Should Know: Fast Focus Study Guide

Search Amazon Kindle books to find other study guides written by

JT Thomas, MD

Internal Medicine Study Guide

Medical Oncology Study Guide

Multiple Myeloma Study Guide

Differential Diagnosis Study Guide

Rheumatology Study Guide